SURVIVING INFLAMMATORY BREAST CANCER

BY
CHARLENE COPELAND

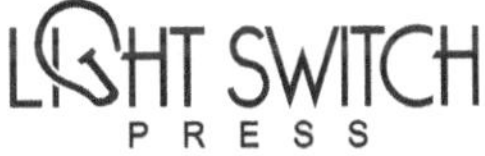

Published by:
Light Switch Press
PO Box 272847
Fort Collins, CO 80527

DEDICATION

I would like to dedicate this book to everyone going through any terminal illness in the past, present, future or have passed away due to an illness, and to the caregivers for giving the time and patience to take care of someone facing terminal illness.

I lost my husband, Bob (lung cancer) in 2002 and my sister, Mary Ann (lung cancer) in 2006.

They were both with me in 1999 and 2000 to see me through my ordeal and I wish I could have done more for them.

My Father, Mother, Father-in Law and Mother-in-Law all passed away from cancer and I have a cousin, Cheryl going through chemo and radiation at the present time.

Both of my brother's, Raymond and Oram had prostate cancer surgery and are fine now.

I pray there will be a cure for all these diseases in the future and please know I will be praying for each and of you.

INTRODUCTION

Readers; before I tell my story, I would like to say something about inflammatory breast cancer.

It is a rare type of breast cancer that develops rapidly, making the affected breast red, swollen and tender. In my case, it looked crinkly and the skin looked thick. My breast was very warm. It looked like an orange peel. It was also itching.

I was told this occurs when the cancer cells block the lymphatic vessels in skin covering the breast. It is considered a locally advanced cancer which means it has spread from the point of origin to nearby tissue and possibly to nearby lymph nodes.

It can easily be confused with a breast infection, which is exactly what my first reaction was. I thought I had been bit by and insect or something. I put antibiotic cream on it and thought it would be fine. Actually a few days later, I thought it was. It looked fine to me. What I didn't know at the time, was that this was going to be the beginning of the greatest change of my life. I didn't have the slightest clue what was to happen in the future.

Fortunately, the doctor noticed something was wrong when I went in for my appointment and sent me for a mammogram right away. In this case though, there is not a lump. A mammogram does not show this type of cancer.

I was lucky to have a sister that was an X-ray technician and was the one to do the mammogram. She left me to put my top back on while she showed the films to the radiologist and I noticed my breast was changing colors. When she came back, I ask her to look at my breast and see what she thought. She decided to see if the doctor would check it before I went home. He came it to check it and he couldn't believe what it was doing. He says, "I have never seen anything like this before. There is something wrong; but I don't think it is cancer. I am going to refer you for a biopsy, just to be on the safe side."

The next week I had the biopsy and when the result came back, it was positive for cancer.

NO

MY STORY STARTING WITH THE SYMPTOMS

When I got out of bed on the morning of 2 July 1999, I knew something was wrong with my right breast. It felt hot and was itching and burning.

I walked into the bathroom and took my gown off, I noticed my breast was red, crinkly, and warm to the touch. It looked like and orange peel. I first thought I had been bit by an insect and it would be fine. After taking a shower, I rubbed an antibiotic cream on it which helped ease the burning and itching.

My husband, Bob thought I should go to the emergency room; but I had an appointment to see my doctor on July 12. I told him I would just try to wait until that appointment. The appointment had originally been for July 2; but the doctor's office had called and re-scheduled due to the doctor being out of town.

Our son, Bob was flying home from California that afternoon with his wife, her father, mother and aunt. They were coming home for the family re-union on my side of the family.

Life was hectic for the next few days and with all the excitement, I never thought about my breast. It bothered me some but; it looked better and I thought it was fine.

DOCTOR APPOINTMENT

On July 12, I went to my doctor's appointment. I was concerned about a cyst on my left breast. The doctor checked it and we discussed removing it. (The cyst was removed a few days later without a problem). Then he examined my right beast and says, "Have you had a problem with your right breast?" I told him what had happened. He says, "There is something wrong with your breast and I want you to get a mammogram as soon as possible. I'll have the nurse see if we can get you in tomorrow." Before I left to go home, I had an appointment for the next morning.

My husband, Bob was with me. We decided to stop by my sister Mary's house on the way home. Mary worked night shift in Radiology. I told her what was going on and that I had an

Appointment for the next morning.

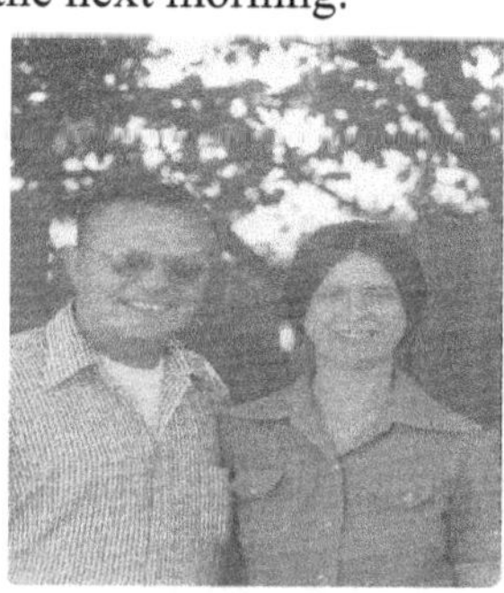

Bob and me

MAMMOGRAM

Later that evening, I received a call from Mary, telling me to come to the hospital. She had talked to Dr. Runyon, the Radiologist and he told her to call and have me come in and not wait until the next morning. She was to do the mammogram and he was going to read it before going home.

When I arrived, Mary did the mammogram and Dr. Runyon read it. She came back to tell me he didn't see anything to be concerned with. I said, "Mary look at my breast? It is changing colors." It would be pinkish, turn beige, blue and back to pink. She looked at it and says, "Let me see if Dr. Runyon will come look at this." He came in and couldn't believe his eyes. He says, "I have never seen a breast change color like this before. I don't think it is anything to be concerned with; but I will refer you for a biopsy just to be on the safe side."

I was scheduled for a biopsy on July 26 and sure enough when the result came back in August, I was told by Dr. Walthal that I had breast cancer. Dr. Walthal was the one that did the biopsy. She told me that she had not expected the result to be positive. I was told on Friday and an appointment was made for me on Monday, August 16 to see Dr. Patrick Gomez at St. John's in Springfield, Missouri.

APPOINTMENT WITH DOCTOR GOMEZ

My husband, Bob and niece Coan accompanied me to my appointment. I was still in shock and couldn't believe this happening to me. My first impression of Doctor

Gomez wasn't very favorable. He came in and says "You have inflammatory breast cancer. It is an aggressive cancer and you probably only have at the maximum six months to live." He left the room. I think I went into shock. I turned to Bob and Coan and said, "I guess I am going to die." For some reason, I couldn't cry even though I felt like it. Dr. Gomez came back in the room a few minutes later and told us he would explain everything, now that the initial shock was over.

He first explained to me exactly what inflammatory breast cancer was and that I would be getting eight very strong chemo treatments, wait a month and have a mastectomy. I would wait another month to take six and one-half weeks of radiation treatments. Chemo had to be first so the cancer wouldn't spread. This treatment was my only hope. If it didn't work, there wasn't anything that could be done.

While he was out of the room, I had read a poster on his wall saying to eat your fruits and vegetables, don't drink, smoke, etc. It was everything you could do to prevent cancer. I had done all that, so I ask him, "If I have done all this, how come I have cancer?" He says, "Charlene, I can't answer that. I don't know."

I left for home that day praying to God to see me through the next months

CHEMO TREATMENTS

My first chemo treatment was scheduled for August 18. I received it by IV. I would be scheduled for surgery the following week to have a port inserted.

The treatment was going to be Cyclophosphamide and Taxotere which would take five hours followed by another ten minutes of Adriamycin (nickname Big Red). I was given something to drink and snack on during the treatment and for my ride home. I was advised I may lose my hair in about 2 weeks. That proved to be true. Exactly two weeks and I woke up one morning with my hair left on my pillow. What was left attached to my scalp was coming out by the handful. My hair was long. It reached the middle of my back, Bob cut the remaining long strands off and shaved my head. That wasn't the most devastating to me though. I also lost the hair on my whole body, even my eye brows and lashes. The only good part was, my legs and underarms wouldn't need to be shaved anymore. Thanks to the American Cancer Society, I was able to borrow two wigs for use until my hair grew back. They were returned when no longer needed, so another cancer patient could use them. When I went for chemo, they had a box of donated head coverings, caps and scarves, that you could go through and take what you needed. I usually wore a cap or scarf because wearing a wig on a bald head doesn't work very well. It didn't for me anyway. There isn't anything to pin the wig to. I had one on one day when I went for chemo and when I got out of the car in the parking lot, it was sideways on my head!

August 23, Bob took me to the hospital for a Neupogen (Filgrastrim) shot. It is given to the patient to help the body make white blood cells after taking chemo. It can also improve survival in people who have been exposed to radiation. I was to get one a day for seven days. I took it again on August 24; but on August 25, they could not give me a shot due to swelling of my arm. They called Dr. Gomez and he told them to not give me anymore shots. I was allergic.

It took about four days after the chemo before I felt nauseous and that lasted for about one and one-half weeks. When I started feeling like I was back with the living it was time to go for the next treatment. Oh, did I ever dread going in for the treatment, knowing how sick I would be.

I had a port for my second treatment on September 15. My blood and port were checked before the treatment. Everything went well. The third treatment on October 6 and fourth on October 28 were given without any problem; but for the fifth on November 18, the port was blocked; but they were finally able to get it cleared in time for my treatment.

I was given medicine for nausea and to help me sleep. I was also given a pill to take on day ten instead of taking the Neupogen shot.

In between treatments was always the same. I felt good for the first few days and then I would wake up one morning so sick I was crawling to the bathroom. I felt like I was going to die any moment. It was a feeling I will never forget. My mouth always felt like it was full of salt. I would rinse with water and it seemed like it got worse instead of better. Eating potato chips was the only thing that helped. Why potato chips, I don't know since they are salty; but it worked. Most patients have a sweet taste, so I was told the salty taste is unusual. But; I guess, I am unusual.

About half way through my chemo treatments, my son, Bob came home for a surprise visit. My brother, Oram lives in Illinois. He picked Bob up at the airport in St. Louis and stopped in Sullivan, Missouri to get Raymond, our brother. They all three spent the weekend with us. My sister, Mary and her husband, John came over to our house Saturday afternoon. I was sitting on the front porch watching all of them in our front yard talking. I was out of it, sitting there zoned out. I got up several times and went in the house. My sister, Mary realized I wasn't acting right, so she came to see what I was doing. I had a bottle of pills in my hand. She wanted to know what I was doing. I told her I didn't feel well and needed more medicine. She realized that I had been going in the house to take medicine and that is why I was zoned out. It was like that on my worst days. I felt so bad, I didn't realize what I was doing at times.

When I went in for my sixth treatment in December, my port was blocked, they couldn't get it cleared to give the treatment. I was sent to the hospital to have dye put through it to see where the blockage was. When I was finished, I was told I could go home.

Dr. Gomez had told me to come back to see him before I made the hour drive home. When I arrived at his office, I was told he had gone home for the day. On the drive home, a storm came up, lightning, thunder and lots of rain. Unlocking the front door, we heard our phone ringing. It was Dr. Gomez wanting to know where I was. I told him I had just gotten home. He says, "I thought I told you to check with me before leaving." I say, "I did. I was told you had gone home. I ask the receptionist to check and make sure because you told me to check back with you. She said it wouldn't do any good because you were not back there." He says, "Get back up here as soon as possible, you have a blood clot and I want you in the hospital as soon as possible." He asked to talk to my husband and when Bob hung up the phone, he says, "grab a bag with a few things, we are going back to the hospital and the doctor is meeting us in emergency. He said, he knows it is storming out; for me to drive carefully. If that blood clot breaks loose, you are in trouble."

When we arrived at the hospital, Dr. Gomez met us and I was admitted and taken directly to a room, IV put in and put on Heparin.

As soon as the blood clot was taken care of, Dr. Gomez came in to see me one morning and says, "As soon as I find a surgeon, you will be scheduled for surgery and get that port taken out. It will probably be sometime today." I jokingly replied, "Dr. Gomez, you don't have to go out on the street to find a surgeon, do you?" He laughed and said, "I hope not." It was late in the evening before they finally took me to surgery. Taking the port out was an experience. To get it to pop out, they had me standing on my head. When it came out, it flew across the room. We were all laughing. I didn't get back to my room until about 11:00 p.m. I was surprised to see my sister, Mary waiting for me.

I hadn't had anything to eat all day and when they brought me some food, I couldn't eat. When I tried, it came right back up. By morning, I was starving. I was anxiously waiting for breakfast and when it showed up it was liquids. I ask the nurse, "What happened to my breakfast?" She says, "You are scheduled for surgery today and can't have anything solid to eat."

I say, "I had surgery last night, I am starving." She says, "Let me check your records." A few minutes later, a huge breakfast was delivered to me with an apology.

My stay in the hospital was ten days and I was given my sixth chemo treatment before I was released to go home.

The staff didn't want me to leave. They had gotten use to my husband coming in for daily visits. Sometimes he came in twice even though it was an hour drive from Sleeper to Springfield. I guess he just wanted something to do. They always had a good time with him. He kept the coffee going in the visiting area!

During my stay in the hospital, one of the nurses asked me if I was going to have reconstructive surgery. I told her no. She says, "Why not? It would probably make you feel better. You should think about it." When Dr. Gomez talked to me about my surgery and what they were going to do, he didn't mention it. I asked him, "Is it possible for me to have reconstructive surgery when they remove my breast?" He says, "Where did you get that idea? The answer is no. You are not a candidate for reconstructive surgery because of the type of cancer you have." He explained the reason was they needed to be able to treat me immediately if my cancer came back. I learned that day that you should be careful when talking to someone about their medical problem. You can get their hopes up just to be let down.

I had two more chemo treatments to take after my hospital stay and they were given by IV. My seventh treatment was given on January 7, 2000 and the eighth and last January 28.

I had to wait thirty days before the mastectomy. It was scheduled for March 6.

MASTECTOMY

My brother, Raymond and sister, Alice spent the night at our house on March 5 and went to the hospital the morning of March 6 with us. I was admitted to St. John's Hospital in Lebanon, Missouri for the procedure. Dr. Walthal was doing the surgery. It was a long day for my family. I was in surgery about five hours.

When I was released to go home, I had two drains (one on each side) and so many staples that I felt like a board. Bob had taken a pillow, so I could hold it against my chest on the ride home. We lived on a gravel road and the ride was bumpy. The pillow didn't help much; but I was still thankful for it.

I had to milk the drains into a container I was given. Thanks to my sister, Mary. She came by the house on her way to work every day to check on me. She made sure they were drained properly and gave me a shot in the stomach that I had to take every day.

Mary was concerned on March 12 when she arrived. My right arm was swollen and she thought I should go to the emergency room. She knew Dr. Walthal was going to be on duty. Bob and I told her I would come in later to the hospital. When we arrived, Mary met us at the emergency room. She had already told Dr. Walthal about my arm. While I was in the exam room, I will never forget Bob and Dr. Walthal acting like chickens to cheer me up. They were hilarious. How many doctors would do that for a patient?

I was admitted to the hospital and the next morning had a Cat Scan. I had lymphedema and ended up for a three day stay. The evening before I was released, Dr. Walthal removed the left drain and the morning I was released she removed the right one. Having a drain pulled out is not fun. It hurts!!! Dr. Walthal was cool though and got my mind off what she was doing while she pulled it out. She was an expert at pulling your attention away from what she was doing. What a special doctor.

Now, my next step was lymphedema treatments. Oh, what fun.

LYMPHEDEMA AND RADIATION TREATMENTS

I had to go to St. John's Hospital in Springfield, Missouri for Lymphedema treatments. I started them on March 27. I took the treatments Monday through Friday. I had massage therapy every day and on Tuesday and Thursday I had to get in the pool. I learned how to massage and wrap my arm. It was unwrapped in the morning and wrapped before I went home. I had to keep my arm wrapped over the weekend. They gave me a video tape on how to wrap and massage your arm to take home and watch over the weekend. They only had one tape, so I recorded eight more for them that weekend. By the time I had them recorded, I had memorized everything.

I had a total of twenty treatments. The last one was April 21.

I was marked for radiation while I was still taking Lymphedema treatments and that was tricky. How can you be careful and not wash the markings off until they get your three molds made? No matter how careful you try to be, the markings still get washed off and you need to be marked again. It wasn't my fault; but they still weren't happy.

My radiation started April 10 and after twenty-five treatments ended on May 12. What a Mother's Day gift!

The day of my last treatment, I was happy that I wasn't very red and not too burnt. Dr. Rodger's says, "Just wait for a few days. The radiation hasn't stopped working yet." He was right. A few days later, I looked like a piece of partially fried bacon. My right chest was blistered and when the blisters broke, I was raw. They had given me Aquaphor; but that didn't help. I was miserable. I finally tried Aloe Vera. I would slit the leaves and lay them on my chest. My sister, Mary had a friend, Sally that gave me several Aloe Vera plants. Thank God for Sally. She was a life saver. It does work. (The next time I went to Radiation, I told them about the Aloe Vera and a few years later, I was in the hospital with Mary and stopped by to see them. I was told, they now get donations of Aloe Vera plants for the patients.)

I took some white t-shirts and cut them down the front. I cut holes on both sides and tied them with a shoe string. I couldn't stand anything touching my chest. Most of the time I just left the t-shirt open. When company came, I would loosely tie it.

I suffered for three weeks. I sat on the steps of our back porch and cried. I would often ask God to just take me. I was tired of suffering. I finally started to heal. By the end of June, I started feeling more like my old self.

It was only my chest that was burnt, so now when I hear of someone being severely burned, my heart goes out to them

GOING BACK TO WORK

The end of June, I received a call from Ft. Leonard Wood to interview for a job. I told them I was just getting over my cancer and wasn't sure if I should go to work or not. The lady on the phone told me to come on in, maybe we could work something out as it was a temporary position. I had been on the list for a position for three years, so didn't want to turn the opportunity down. I went for the interview, got the position and went to work in July 2000. I

enjoyed my time working at the fort. My co-workers knew that I had just gone through cancer treatment and they helped me come out of my shell and not be depressed.

I worked until January 2001 and I decided to retire. I had been a federal worker before, so had time accrued. The job was still available; but I decided I needed some time to recuperate.

About four months later, I was called and told the employee that had taken my position had left to go back to their old position and would I be interested in coming back to work for about six months. I had to interview again and go out of retirement; but I decided to go back. They had a party for me when I returned. We were all happy to see each other. I couldn't ask for better co-workers. I worked until January 2002. This time my retirement was for good.

CANCER COMES
BACK IN NECK

In February 2002, I fell and jammed my collarbone, of all things; running from a rooster!

I went to my primary care physician and he gave me a prescription for amoxicillin. I took it as prescribed. My collarbone still bothered me, but I thought it would be alright.

The end of April, Bob and I took a road trip to Glendale, California to visit our son Bob and his wife, Martha. In May, over the Memorial Day week we took another trip to Billings, Montana in our motorhome to take my nephew and his wife to a bowling conference.

The first part of June, Bob and I had doctor's appointments. On his visit, he found out he had lung cancer and would need surgery. When I went to see Doctor Gomez, he took one look at my neck and ask me what happened, did I go to the doctor and what did I take for it. When I told him, he looked at me and says, "Your cancer is back." He walked out of the room and came back a few minutes later telling me I have an appointment over at the Fremont building now for a needle biopsy. I left his office and went for the biopsy.

When the results came back, I went for an appointment with Doctor Gomez. They had notified him that it was positive, but he didn't have the results in my records. When he called to get them, they couldn't find them. He was not happy. He scheduled me for surgery to have a biopsy within a few days. They removed several lymph nodes at the time. Another six and a half weeks of radiation were going to be necessary.

Two weeks later, Bob was hospitalized with pancreatitis. In another couple weeks, he ended up at the emergency room and needed emergency surgery for gangrene of the small intestine. They removed a few inches of his small intestine. Two weeks later he was hospitalized for lung surgery. Life seemed to be spiraling out of control.

HUSBAND HAS LUNG SURGERY AND I START RADIATION FOR SECOND TIME

On August 16, 2002, we picked our son up at the Springfield Airport. We spent an enjoyable weekend with him. On Monday morning we all three went to the hospital for Bob's pre-op and my first radiation treatment. That evening we went out to eat with friends. The next morning, we had Bob at the hospital at 6:00 a.m. for surgery.

While he was in surgery, I got a radiation treatment. When I arrived back to the waiting room, they had already told our son that he was out of surgery and in the recovery room. The surgery had gone fine and we would be able to see him in a few minutes. The next thing we knew, they were bringing him out of recovery and putting him in a room. The nurse was not happy as his blood pressure was low and they couldn't get it stabilized.

Once it was stabilized, we were able to visit him. We stayed until visiting hours were over the first night.

Wednesday, Thursday and Friday, we visited Bob and I would get my radiation treatment. While I went for my radiation treatment at

1:00 p.m., our son stayed with his dad. We never left for home until late in the evening. We spent as much time as possible with Bob.

Saturday, August 24, 2002, Bob was released to go home and the next morning, he passed away on the kitchen floor.

That afternoon, I had to go to the funeral home for arrangements for his funeral. Monday morning, I went for radiation. His viewing was in the evening and Tuesday morning the funeral services. I didn't go for radiation the day of the funeral; but Wednesday I went for radiation. I wanted to get it over; although they said I could take the rest of the week off and make up at the end.

After everyone left for home, my niece, Coan stayed with me, so I wouldn't be alone. Every day, Monday through Friday, we made the trip to Springfield for my radiation treatment. One of our trips in the Winter, there was snow and ice on the road and on our way to Springfield, I hit a slick spot in the road and my car did a complete turn in a circle on the freeway. There was a car behind me that slowed down when he saw what had happened. When I was going straight again, he passed and gave me a thumbs up! We both thought we were done for. Thanks to God, we didn't end up in an accident. She spent nine months with me. I don't know what I would have done without her. She has a special place in my heart for all she has done for me. Thank you, Coan!

After radiation, Doctor Gomez wanted me to take Herceptin, but I refused. He asked me to think about it until my next appointment. When I went back, he said he had an option for me. There was a chemo pill called Xeloda. It wouldn't make me as sick and my hair wouldn't fall out. I would have to take it the rest of my life. I wouldn't take it every day. I would be on so many days; off so many days. I decided I would go with this option. I was on Xeloda for nine years. I continued seeing Dr. Gomez until 2005.

I sold my home in Sleeper, Missouri in May 2004 and moved to Sullivan, Missouri. I wanted to keep Dr. Gomez as my oncologist, but the drive from Sullivan to Springfield got to be too much so Dr. Gomez referred me to Dr. Bond in Rolla, Missouri.

TREATMENT FROM 2005 UNTIL PRESENT

I was under Dr. Bond's care until 2011. During this period, I had three biopsies on my left breast. All three were benign. The first and last were surgery; but I was talked into getting the needle biopsy for the second one. Never again will I do that. It was uncomfortable and hurt. After the third one, I told the doctor I wouldn't have any more biopsies on my left breast. He told me there are other options. I hope so!

I also had a brain scan and was told there was a spot on my right side near my temple which we needed to keep an eye on. I also had to have the big toe nail on my right foot removed because of fungus.

In 2011, I transferred to Missouri Baptist Hospital in Sullivan, Missouri. My first appointment, I was scheduled for an appointment at Barnes in St. Louis for a PET Scan. When the results came back, I was told my cancer was back in my clavicle and they wanted me to go in the following week to have a port put in and start chemo. I refused the port and chemo. No way was I going through that again.

I continued taking the Xeloda until 2012. I got hand and foot syndrome where my hands and feet were peeling until they would bleed. At this time, I also started having spells where I would start feeling sick. First my mouth would get warm like I was going to throw up and I would start shaking so bad that my teeth chattered. I would take

Ibuprophen, go to bed, curl up in a ball and wonder if I would make it. I usually fell asleep and when I woke up, I would be alright.

In 2014, I purchased a home in Cuba, Missouri where I now live. I continue to see the oncologist once a year. I no longer have a problem with the hand and foot syndrome. The last time I had the shaking spell was about five years ago. Where I had the radiation on my right side of my chest still bothers me. It stings and burns. I have a prosthesis, but I seldom wear it as it bothers the radiated area of my chest. I have a spot near my clavicle that bothers me; but I was told right after I moved that it turned out to be arthritis instead of cancer. That was the first time I had been told that and I wonder what would have happened if I had let them put in the port and start me on chemo for the cancer that hadn't returned. I'm just happy I turned it down.

I have never gained the energy back. I am constantly tired. I take naps twice a day if possible. Some days I get a jolt of energy and want to do everything in one day and the next day I am wiped out! I thank God every day that I am still alive. I know the cancer could come back anytime; but; I have been lucky. It has been almost twenty years since I was first diagnosed. The doctors say I am lucky to be alive and to keep doing whatever I am doing.

I agree. Most of all I thank God for seeing me through every step of the way!

There is one last thing I would like to say before I end my story and that is this, "I have been in conversations where I have been told I should not say "my cancer." We'll it was my cancer. It was in my body. I felt the pain and went through being so sick I wanted to die. I prayed it would go away. I willed it away, but I had to fight and fight hard to still be alive today. Another thing, everyone's cancer is different. What happened to me or what I went through may not be the same as another person. The type of cancer and treatment may be different. Anyway, enough said. I will end my story and again say, thank you, God for watching over me."

ACKNOWLEDGEMENTS

There are so many people to thank for their support during this trying time in my life. Thank God, my husband Bob and sister Mary were still alive. They were my pillars and kept me going. I have since lost them to lung cancer. My son, Bob, thanks for being there during my fight and the death of your father. I don't know what I would do without you. To my sister Alice, brother's Raymond (Butch) and Oram, you were there supporting me always. I love you. Coan, you were by my side through good and bad times. I appreciate all you did. John Blender (Mary's husband) who was always there when I needed help. Rosanna and Chris (Mary's daughter and son). When you were needed, you were always available. Faye, a friend that has gone through a lot in her lifetime and kept me going by giving me pep talks and telling me to hang in there. Faye, you are one of a kind and I thank you from the bottom of my heart.

Dr. Gomez, you are the best. I couldn't have had a better doctor. You are the reason I am here to write this book. Thanks to Dr. Runyon for referring me for the biopsy, Dr. Walthal for the surgeries and great care. Dr. Rodgers and his staff for the great burn you gave me in radiation! You did a wonderful job even if it hurt.

Thanks to all in the medical field that had anything to do with my treatment. You saved my life and I am forever grateful.

Thanks to the American Cancer Society for wigs and refund for some of my gas to get to treatments. To the donors giving of their time to make head coverings for chemo patients. Thanks to the cancer group at St. John's in Lebanon for all the free boost to keep me going.

Thanks again everyone, you are the best. I will never forget.

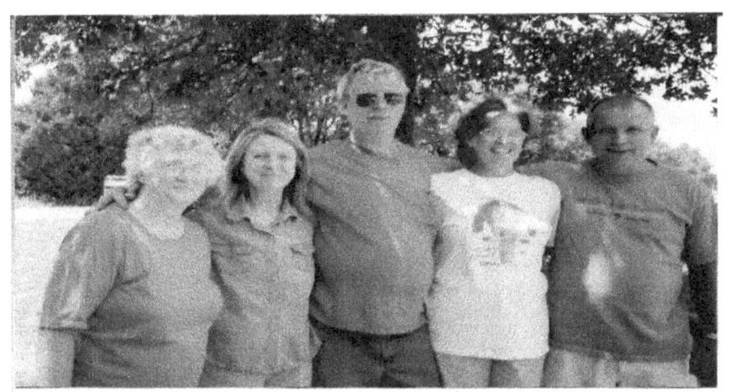

My sister Alice, me, brother (Raymond), sister Mary and brother (Oram)

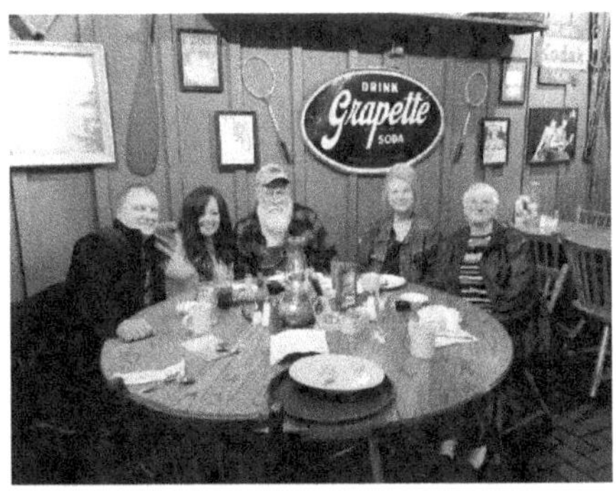

My son Bob, wife Martha, Dave, me and Alice (2019)

THE END

www.ingramcontent.com/pod-product-compliance
Lightning Source LLC
Chambersburg PA
CBHW050806240726

48654CB00008B/660